Neck Pain

Neck Pain: Common Causes and Home Treatment

By JC Scout

Introduction

The neck is an important part of your body. It supports your head and allows you to move it in various directions. It is also responsible for protecting the nerves that relay motor and sensory information from your brain to other parts of your body. Moreover, the neck houses the arteries that do the important work of supplying blood to the brain right from the heart.

As such, if the neck is in pain, you'll find it very difficult to function properly as you go about your day.

Unfortunately, neck pain is quite common in today's world. Researchers estimate that nearly 7 out of 10 people experience neck pain at some point in their lives. However, knowing that others experience neck pain does little to alleviate your own pain.

You want answers to all the questions that may be running through your mind right now.

For instance, you may have questions like:

Why does the neck hurt so much?

What causes this pain?

What can you do to ease the pain?

How can you make sure it does not happen again?

And many others.

This book seeks to answer these and any other questions you may have about neck pain to ensure at the end of it, you take measures to alleviate the pain and possibly prevent it from recurring.

Read along to discover what neck pain is, why your neck hurts and what you can do to treat neck pain.

Let's begin.

Thanks again for purchasing this book. I hope you enjoy it!

information is without contract or any type of guarantee assurance.

The trademarks that are used are without any consent, and the publication of the trademark is without permission or backing by the trademark owner. All trademarks and brands within this book are for clarifying purposes only and are the owned by the owners themselves, not affiliated with this document.

Table of Contents

Chapter 1: What Is Neck Pain?

Of course, you know when you experience neck pain but what actually is it?

Well, in order to understand what neck pain is, you need to know how your neck is structured. The first thing to note is that the neck is part of the backbone or spinal column. It consists of seven bones or vertebrae. These vertebrae are separated by intervertebral discs, which absorb shock between the seven bones when you perform various activities and allow your spine to move freely.

Any injury, abnormalities or inflammation to the muscles, bones and ligaments that are found in your neck area results in what is collectively known as neck pain. Neck pain comes in various shapes and sizes.

Neck pain symptoms include:

- Muscle pain – This is where you experience aches and soreness in your neck and shoulder muscles. Your neck may develop a 'crick' or hard knots. These knots are usually tender to the touch and you may feel increased pain if they are pressed.

- Muscle spasm – Muscle spasms are characterized by sudden tightening of the neck muscles. Your neck may feel tight and knotted and you may find it difficult to turn your head. A lot of times, when people wake up with a stiff neck, they have likely experienced muscle spasms. Muscle spasms vary in intensity. They can be painful but the tightening usually goes away quickly.

- Headache – It's not unusual to experience neck-related headaches when your neck is hurting. Such headaches are usually felt in the upper neck or in the back of the head. They are often described as a dull aching and may be accompanied by a stiff or tender neck. If you experience neck-related headaches, you may find yourself feeling worse whenever you move your neck.

- General soreness - Some neck pains fall under general soreness. The pain is mostly situated in one area or spot on the neck. It is tender rather than sharp. Your neck aches but not enough to send you into panic mode.

- Stiff neck – This is where soreness is accompanied by a lack of range in motion. You'll have difficulty moving or turning your head from one side to another. Your neck may feel sore and inflamed.

- Tingling or weakness – You may feel tingling sensations that go beyond the neck and into the shoulders, arms or fingers. These sensations are usually like being pierced with 'pins-and-needles'. They often radiate down one arm instead of both arms. What's more, the tingling sensation may be accompanied by weakness.

- Radiating pain – This is the type of pain attributed to nerve pain. It comes about due to the pinching or irritation of the spinal nerve. It results in a sharp pain that runs along the neck into the shoulders and down the arms. This radiating pain varies in its intensity and can turn into a searing or burning pain. It can shoot through your arm every now and then and then disappear for a while before showing itself again.

- Trouble with gripping – Neck pain can make it difficult for you to grip or lift objects. This is especially so if it is accompanied by numbness, weakness or tingling in the fingers. The weakness may come suddenly and you may find yourself dropping whatever it is you were holding.

As you can see, neck pain symptoms are varied. However, they may end up interfering with your daily activities if they progress. You may find it difficult to do simple tasks such as getting dressed or driving. The severity of the pain may prevent you from working or socializing with others. In other words, neck pain, no matter the intensity, affects the quality of your life. This is why you need to deal with it as soon as possible.

But before you treat it, it would help to know why your neck hurts in the first place.

Chapter 2: Causes Of Neck Pain

There are few things as uncomfortable as being in pain without understanding where the pain comes from. Think about it; if you are unaware of what is causing you pain, you may just end up in the same situation because there's little you can do to prevent the pain. However, if you know the source of pain, you can take measures to treat it and prevent it from coming up in future.

To help you treat and possibly prevent neck pain, let's discuss some of the different causes of neck pain.

Muscle strain

Muscle strain usually occurs when a muscle is torn or overstretched. Muscle strains are common in the neck, shoulder, lower back and hamstring but they can occur in any muscle. If you strain your neck muscles, you may experience symptoms such as:

- Limited range of movement

- Muscle spasms

- Soreness

- Stiffness

- Weakness

- Sudden pain

- Bruising or discoloration

- Knotted-up feeling

Muscle strain is often brought about due to poor flexibility, poor conditioning, failure to warm up properly before exercise or physical activity, fatigue and overexertion. If you suddenly use 'cold muscles' without warming up first, you increase the risk of straining your muscles.

Muscle strain can also be brought about by poor posture. For example, your sleeping position can result in pain and stiffness in the neck, back or shoulders. Things such as the firmness of your mattress, the number of pillows you use and your sleeping position affect the way you feel when you wake up in the morning. If you fall asleep in a bad position, your neck will move out of alignment and this will put a strain on the muscles and lead to soreness in the neck.

Slipped disc

Slipped disc, also known as bulging disc or herniated disc, occurs when the outer layer of your disc ruptures. This exposes the gel-like center of the cervical disc to your spinal nerves and ends up irritating such nerves.

Once the spinal nerves are irritated or inflamed, you feel pain. Pain also occurs due to the swelling that occurs as the jelly-like structure presses into your spinal nerves. A herniated disc may cause radiating pain that goes down your arm and hand. It may also cause pain near the shoulder blade.

So, what causes discs to herniated or bulge?

Well, things like age, improper lifting and injury may all cause your discs to bulge. As you grow older, the discs in your body dry out. They become harder. As a result, the outer wall may weaken. This makes it easier for the gel-like nucleus to tear through the outer wall and when it does, it touches a nerve and causes pain.

People who play sports such as basketball or other contact sports or who are involved in physically challenging occupational activities may have early disc degeneration and as such are at a higher risk of experiencing pain due to a herniated disc.

Degeneration

As you grow older, the discs and vertebrae in the neck start to wear down. You may experience pain in the neck as they degenerate. But apart from age, there are other conditions that can cause discs and vertebrae to generate. These include:

- Inflammation

- Cervical fractures

- Pinched nerves and

- Cervical disc degeneration

Degeneration may lead to chronic or persistent pain. As such, it is important to know how to treat neck pain so as to find some relief.

Cervical spondylosis

Cervical spondylosis is a degeneration that affects the spinal discs in your neck. It is also referred to as degenerative arthritis or osteoarthritis. A lot of people who suffer from the condition do not exhibit any symptoms. But when symptoms occur, they usually include stiffness and pain in the neck region.

Cervical spondylosis may cause the space needed by your nerve roots and spinal cord to narrow. This may cause the nerve roots or spinal cord to become pinched. In this case, you may experience symptoms such as:

- A lack of coordination

- Difficulty walking

- Tingling and numbness in the arms, hands or feet

- Weakness in your arms or legs and

- Loss of bowel control

Cervical spondylosis worsens with age and is common in people over 60 years of age.

Whiplash

Whiplash is a form of neck strain. It occurs when your neck moves forwards and the backwards very quickly to resemble the cracking of a whip. The sudden force damages the tendons and muscles in your neck. It may come with symptoms such as:

- Tightness in the neck -the muscles may feel hardened or knotted.

- Pain when moving your head

- Tenderness

- Headaches – the headaches usually start at the base of your skull and move towards your forehead.

- Decreased range of motion

Whiplash is common among those who suffer car accidents but it can afflict those who play contact sports such as football. Basically, any movement that causes your neck to move quickly back and forth may cause whiplash.

But there's something important to note.

The effects of whiplash don't have to be felt immediately. You may feel such effects within hours or within days. Thus, you have to be on the lookout for neck strains whenever you experience sudden movements. Also, it is good to note that whiplash is often accompanied by concussion. If you notice symptoms such as nausea, dizziness, trouble talking, confusion or excessive sleepiness, it would be best to seek medical care.

Stress and anxiety

Stress is linked to a number of physical symptoms including neck pain. Here's the thing. When you are stressed, you may tense up. This causes the muscles in your neck to tighten and as a result, you end up feeling pain.

Stress leads to the famous fight or flight response. This increases the adrenaline in your body to prepare your body for action. Your blood pressure heightens, your blood supply increases and the muscles surrounding your spine tense up and spasm in preparation for whatever action you want to take.

However, if no action is taken, the stress is felt on your neck and shoulders. You may feel like the 'weight of the world' is on your shoulders. This is why a lot of people who are stressed complain about neck pain especially when their stress level goes up.

Unfortunately, stress is also linked to increased pain and depression. This means stress can cause your neck and shoulder muscles to tense up and this leads to pain. In turn, the pain you experience can put you in a worse mood and lead you to experience more pain, which adds on to your stress. In simpler terms, stress not only contributes to pain but it can also cause you to feel increased pain resulting in a vicious cycle.

Can't decide if your neck pain is associated with stress? Do this one simple thing. Journal. Start journaling when you have exacerbations of your neck pain, do you have a headache associated with your neck pain? What happened on that day? Did you have a stressful work meeting or a fight with your spouse? Was it a hard day with the kids or were you worried about bills? If you start to see a trend, then your neck pain is associated with stress and it will be easier in many ways to treat.

Non-specific neck pain

Sometimes the cause of neck pain cannot be pinpointed. You may hurt your neck without being able to identify how you did it. Non-specific neck pain often arises due to minor tear or sprain to the muscle tissue. It is a common type of neck pain.

But it's good to note that non-specific neck pain may occur due to poor posture. If you spend a lot of time sitting at a desk or bending forward, your neck may come out of alignment for long periods of time and this places a strain on the muscles. Later on, you may move in a certain way that causes pain and you may fail to pinpoint where the pain stems from. In truth, the muscle strain built up over time. It didn't just occur from nowhere. There are times when you will wake up and have neck pain and cannot associate it with an injury or a trauma.

Neck Pain and Sleep

In recent years there have been a number of studies that have shown an increase in the correlation between the quality and quantity of sleep and its relationship to pain. So, there is increasing evidence that poor sleep will increase your pain. It is also proven that pain will disrupt sleep, thus compounding the pain/sleep cycle. However, the literature suggests that the effect of sleep on pain is greater than that of pain on sleep. In fact, there is growing evidence that poor sleep habits can compound the pain experience leading to increased pain even in those who do not normally have pain. Therefore, it is extremely important to maintain a healthy sleep pattern known as sleep hygiene. This is important in regulating normal physiological process to decrease pain. This also allows tissue to heal.

•	Maintain healthy sleep habits

•	If you have poor sleep habits, create a routine around bedtime and try to follow it.

•	Complete relaxation techniques prior to going to bed to aid with sleep.

•	Understand that your dysfunction in sleep can also lead to a decrease in pain pressure threshold.

•	Seek help from your doctor if poor sleep is affecting your pain.

Yes, there are several causes of neck pain. But whatever the cause, you need to deal with the pain in order to find relief. Fortunately, there are various treatments and tricks you can use to get rid of neck pain. Let us look at some of them.

Chapter 3: Neck Pain Treatment

Your neck is very important to movement but it is also delicate. When it is hurting, you want to treat it in a way that will get rid of pain, not make things worse. As such, you must treat it gently. You can use different strategies to lessen neck pain, some of which include:

Ice pack

In the world of sports, ice therapy is commonly used in the case of injury, sprain or strain. This is because it works well in reducing inflammatory responses, cooling superficial tissues, reducing pain, decreasing hypoxic cell death and reducing edema formation. Ice not only reduces inflammation but also speeds up healing.

You can use ice therapy for neck pain relief. In order to do so, you should:

- Crush some ice cubes and place them in a plastic bag.

- Place the plastic bath on a thin towel and wrap it up.

- Place the wrap on the injured area for about 15 minutes at a time.

- Repeat the treatment every 2 to 3 hours within a 24-hour period.

The ice should not be applied to your skin directly. In fact, instead of placing the ice pack in one area, you can engage in a form of ice massage - an ice massager can make your work easier. You can use it to massage your neck and find relief from pain. When applying ice massage, you should hold the ice in one spot for less than 3 minutes at a time and then move on to a different spot.

If you do not have an ice massager, you can make one by freezing water in a paper cup or a foam cup. Once done, tear the top off and proceed to rub the ice on your neck. Ensure that you move the ice before 3 minutes are up.

Hydrotherapy

When your neck hurts, you want to find relief. One way you can do this is by doing some stretching exercises. Unfortunately, such exercises can prove very painful depending on the extent of your injury. This is where hydrotherapy comes in.

Hydrotherapy or water therapy comes in handy when you want to exercise the neck without aggravating the injury. This is because water has certain properties that make it easier for you to exercise. One of the properties is **buoyancy**. When you exercise in water, you don't feel the effects of gravity as much as you would if you exercise on land. Water helps support your weight and enables you to move in various positions simply because it eliminates the gravitational forces. You can lift your limbs and turn from side to side without using a lot of effort.

Another property water has is **viscosity**. This means that it provides resistance by means of gentle friction. This allows you to strengthen and condition your muscles while greatly reducing the risk of further injury. Water also helps reduce the perception of pain. It provides a relaxing atmosphere and warmth that aide in healing.

One simple exercise you can do in a pool of water is the clock exercise. This is where you move your right leg forward in a lunge position and straighten your hands forwards in line with your shoulders. The idea is to keep one hand stationary as you move the other hand and your neck as the hand of a clock would move in both directions. Repeat the exercise 9-15 times as it gets easier and remember to be very gentle in your movements.

Keep in mind that you don't need a pool in order to benefit from hydrotherapy. You can easily engage in water therapy in your shower. In order to do this, you should allow warm water to target the affected neck area for 3 to 4 minutes. Once the time is up, switch to cold water and allow the water to target the area for 30 to 60 seconds before switching back to warm water. Repeat the process again and again. The warm water does the important job of increasing blood circulation and the cold water works to reduce inflammation and give you relief from pain.

Epsom salt bath

An Epsom salt bath is useful in reducing stress, relieving muscle tension and relieving pain. Epsom salt contains magnesium sulfate. Magnesium sulfate is known as a natural muscle relaxant. It also helps reduce pain and swelling.

In order to prepare an Epsom salt bath, you should:

- Prepare a warm bath and add 1 to 2 cups of the salt in the water.

- Soak in the water and target the neck area for 15 to 20 minutes.

- Repeat the process daily until you neck heals completely.

If you suffer from issues such as diabetes, high blood pressure or heart issues, you should avoid this remedy and stick to water therapy.

Massage therapy

As you've seen, there are various things that can cause neck pain. Some things such as posture can be difficult to correct all the time. For example, you may spend long hours at your desk. As such, you end up getting tired and feeling pain not because of the way you sit but because of how long you sit. A massage can help loosen up your muscles and find relief from pain.

How so?

Well, your neck contains arteries. These arteries are responsible for supplying blood to parts of your brain. When you're forced to sit at your desk for long hours, your neck becomes stiff. This reduces the flow of blood to your brain and it can result in issues such as insomnia, headaches and fatigue. A neck massage does the important work of relieving that stiffness. It opens up the way for your blood to flow freely to the brain.

A neck massage also helps when it comes to the circulation of a fluid known as CSF. This fluid floats in the brain and is responsible for supplying some oxygen and glucose to your brain. If you're experiencing tightness in your neck, the fluid circulation is hindered. This ends ups causing headaches, poor concentration and fatigue. A massage paves way for the fluid to circulate and this improves brain function.

Another good thing about getting a massage is that it helps keep your joints limber. This means that it reduces the chances of you pulling a muscle. Thus, you can enjoy a range of motion throughout the day without the risk of straining your neck.

- Start by taking a hot shower. Once you're done, pat your skin dry.

- Warm up one tablespoon of the massage oil you want to use.

- Gently rub the oil into your neck using circular motions for several minutes.

- Repeat the procedure every morning until your feel relief.

A massage is supposed to give you relief not to cause your more pain. Of course, you may feel a bit of pain if you rub on a hurt spot but the pain should lessen as you continue to massage the spot. It should not be debilitating. If you feel an unusual amount of pain, stop massaging the area immediately.

As you try out the various neck treatments, it is important to remember that your neck is delicate. You have to be careful when dealing with it especially when it is hurting. Select a treatment and take your time to do it correctly and you will find relief from neck pain. The good thing is there are numerous treatments you can use to treat pain.

Transcutaneous Electrical Nerve Stimulator (TENS) Unit

You can treat neck pain with a transcutaneous electrical nerve stimulator (TENS) unit which are now available over the counter and online. These units provide noninvasive drug free pain relief by providing pulses that are sent via pads through the skin along nerve fibers. The pulses suppress the pain signals that are being sent to the brain, thus breaking the pain cycle. It is also thought that the TENS unit encourages the body to secrete endorphins, hormones that cause an analgesic (pain relieving) effect in the brain.

Now let's look at other form of treatments you can use to treat your neck pain.

Chapter 4: Home Remedies To Treat Neck Pain

Home remedies have been in use for generations. They are often passed on from one generation to the next and they are popular due to the fact that they use ingredients that can readily be found in your home. Plus, the fact that they are often passed down by a loved one adds a sentimental value that provides that placebo effect that lessens pain.

When it comes to neck pain, there are some home remedies that have been known to help alleviate the pain. These include:

Cayenne pepper

Cayenne pepper is good at relieving aches and pains because it contains capsaicin, which happens to be an analgesic. It also has anti-inflammatory properties that come in handy when you want to reduce inflammation.

In order to use cayenne pepper, you should:

- Combine 2 tablespoons of lukewarm olive oil with 1 tablespoon of cayenne pepper powder. Mix the ingredients well.

- Once done, scoop up the mixture and rub it onto your neck in circular motions.

- Repeat the procedure twice a day to find relief from sore muscles.

Don't forget to be careful when handling cayenne pepper because it can be quite irritating if you end up inhaling it or if it gets in your nostrils or eyes. Wear protective gloves or wash your hands thoroughly after handling the cayenne powder.

Another alternative is to use a capsaicin cream. This cream contains the analgesic and anti-inflammatory substance that makes it great for pain relief. You can apply the cream 2-3 times a day. Make sure you rub it onto the sore muscles to allow your skin to absorb it.

You can also prepare a capsaicin coconut oil cream. In order to do this, you should:

- Combine 1 cup of coconut oil with 3 tablespoons of cayenne powder.

- Once done, simmer the mixture on low heat until it melts.

- Stir well for 5 minutes then remove from the heat and pour into a bowl. You can whisk using a hand mixer to get a light and fluffy mixture.

- Allow the mixture to firm up.

- Once it cools, massage onto the neck area.

Before applying any mixture onto your neck area, it is good practice to test your reaction to the mixture. You can do this by applying a little bit of the mixture on your hand and waiting for a few minutes to see how you will react to it before applying it on the affected area.

Ginger

Ginger is well known in many households. A nice cup of ginger tea is often used to treat colds and sore throat. You can also use it to relieve pain and inflammation. This is due to its anti-inflammatory and pain-relieving properties. You can make ginger tea if you:

- Combine half an inch of raw ginger and 2 cups of boiling water.

- Allow the mixture to sit for about 5 to 10 minutes.

- Add some lemon juice and honey to taste and drink up to relieve pain.

You can also use ginger topically to reduce pain and inflammation on the affected area. You can do this by making a ginger compress. You can:

- Grate the ginger. It should be enough to get 3 tablespoons.

- Place the grated ginger in a cheese cloth and wrap it up well.

- Place the wrapped ginger in a bowl of hot water for about 30 seconds.

- Allow the cloth to cool a bit and then press it into your neck area for 15 to 20 minutes.

- Repeat the process several times throughout the day to get relief.

Turmeric

Turmeric is known for its color. You can use it to color foods such as rice and tortillas. You can also use it to flavor food. But there is more to it than its taste and color bringing properties. It has medicinal properties that are hard to ignore.

One of the things that give turmeric its medicinal properties is a compound known as curcumin. This is an active ingredient that has powerful anti-inflammatory effects. Inflammation plays an important role in your body when it acts as it should. It helps your body repair damage and fight foreign invaders. However, it can work against us when it becomes chronic. Instead of helping your fight disease, it can cause your body to attack its own tissues. This is why you must reduce inflammation if you want to reduce pain. Turmeric helps you do that.

Turmeric is also a really strong antioxidant. This means that it is capable of protecting your body from free radicals. This reduces diseases and boosts your body's antioxidant defenses. This comes in handy when your body is trying to deal with neck pain. As such, you need to find ways to consume turmeric. You can make it a point to add turmeric to your food but it would be best to drink it if you wish to relieve pain.

Here is how to go about it:

- In a glass of milk, add 1 teaspoon of turmeric powder.

- Once done, heat the mixture for 5 minutes over low heat.

- Remove the mixture from the heat and add a bit of honey and then let the mixture cool.

- Take twice a day to relieve pain.

When using turmeric, you need to be cautious. It can stain your hands or cloths. Thus, don't place it in something you don't want stained.

Blackstrap molasses

Blackstrap molasses should not be overlooked when it comes to relieving neck pain. It is a super food derived from sugarcane and is loaded with various nutrients that allow the body to deal with pain and inflammation. Some vital nutrients it contains include:

Manganese

This antioxidant works to enhance healthy bone structure, helps to create the enzymes needed for bone building and assists in bone metabolism. It is also important to brain and nervous system function. Essentially, manganese keeps your bones healthy and strong. This is vital when it comes to preventing neck pain. Healthy bones are less susceptible to things such as strain and wear and tear.

Iron

Blackstrap molasses contains a healthy dose of iron. This helps in the production of red blood cells and hemoglobin. This in turn helps eradicate fatigue brought on by various causes. When you're tired, it becomes easier to injure yourself. Any product that can get rid of fatigue is valuable in the fight against neck pain.

Copper

Copper is another valuable nutrient in that it contains anti-inflammatory properties. It is especially useful in reducing symptoms of arthritis. It also helps in normal growth and health. As you've seen, one of the causes of neck pain happens to be arthritis. When you suffer from arthritis, your bones and muscles get the brunt of the disease and become susceptible to wear and tear. If helps to keep them healthy and that is what copper does.

Calcium

Calcium is necessary for maintaining strong bones. It also does the admirable job of helping the heat, nerves and muscles to function as they should. When consume foods high in calcium, the chances of hurting yourself decrease. Blackstrap molasses provides you with this nutrient and should be part of your diet in the fight against neck pain.

You can make it a point to add 1 tablespoon of molasses to a glass of warm water. Mix well and drink the mixture twice each day to alleviate pain.

Apple cider vinegar

Apple cider vinegar is another common product found in homes. A lot of recipes make use of it. You too can use it to reduce neck pain. It has anti-inflammatory and antioxidant properties that help combat pain. It is also rich in nutrients and thus, it should come in handy in case the cause of your pain is a lack of nutrients.

In order to use apple cider vinegar, you should:

- Soak a clean towel in 2 tablespoons of apple cider vinegar.

- Once done, apply the towel on the affected neck area and let it rest there for 2 hours twice a day.

- Alternatively, you can add the apple cider vinegar in your bath water. Place two cups of the product in warm water and soak for 15 to 20 minutes each day until the pain disappears.

Yes, there exists various home remedies you can use to relieve neck pain. But as a rule of thumb, test your reaction to the ingredients before using them on the affected area. A small skin patch test would be better than applying something on the affected area and aggravating the pain. Home remedies work really well especially when they are combined with other neck treatments. Thus, you should be determined to find out which home remedies you prefer.

Apart from using neck treatments and home remedies, there is a lot you can do to relieve neck pain by adjusting your posture. Let's see what this is about.

Chapter 5: Posture

Posture has to do with the way you hold your body when you are moving and when you are not moving. Your posture when you're moving is known as dynamic posture. It covers things such as bending, walking and running.

Your posture when you are not moving is known as static posture. It covers things such as standing, sleeping and sitting.

The way you hold yourself has a lot to do with the health of your neck and your general health.

Think about this, correct anatomic position of the head and neck is: head up, shoulders back with ears over shoulders. Think about the position you are in currently, is it good or poor posture?

Poor posture can:

- Decrease your flexibility

- Cause back, shoulder and neck pain

- Cause your musculoskeletal system to misalign

- Cause your spine to wear and thus, make it prone to injury

- Affect your joint movement

- Make breathing harder

- Increase the risk of falling by affecting your balance

- Make it hard to digest food

Text Neck Syndrome

Text neck syndrome is a new condition that has developed with the advent of 'screen-time'. In other words, constantly looking down. You may not realize it, but the neck takes repetitive stress every time you look up and down from your phone or tablet. With your head in neutral position, looking straight ahead the neck is carrying 10-12 pounds just with your head alone (standing looking in a mirror).

- At 15 degrees downward direction this increases to 27 pounds

- At 30 degrees downward direction this increases to 40 pounds

- At 45 degrees downward direction this increases to 49 pounds

- 60 degrees downward direction this increases to a whopping 60 pounds of pressure is placed on your neck (chin on chest, how most of us look at our phones).

It's little wonder that poor posture is one of the main causes of neck pain. But fortunately, there are some things you can do to correct your posture.

Let's look at some of them:

How to improve your posture when standing:

- Start by standing up straight and tall

- Make sure your shoulders are back and not bent forwards

- As you stand, pull your stomach in

- Ensure your weight is well placed on the balls of your feet

- Don't strain your head. Instead, keep it level.

- Allow your arms to fall naturally at your sides

- Place your feet shoulder-width apart whenever you stand.

It may take awhile to improve your standing posture but with practice, you'll soon be able to stand properly without thinking too much about it. Any discomfort you feel is short term. Don't let it discourage you. Instead, focus on the relief you'll find due to maintaining proper posture.

What about your posture when sitting?

How to improve your posture when sitting:

Well, as you know, many people spend hours at a desk. This contributes to aches and pains. But there are various things you can do to find relief. You should:

- Plant your feet on the floor -if your feet cannot reach the floor, you should use a footrest.

- Make sure your shoulders are relaxed instead of pulled backwards or rounded up

- Place your elbows at 90 degrees bent and close to your body

- Support your back. If the chair has no backrest, use a pillow to support the natural curve at your lower back.

- Make sure your hips and thighs are parallel to the floor and sit on a well-padded seat whenever possible.

If you're used to slouching, you may have to correct your posture every now and then until you get used to sitting properly.

If you work on a computer, you should ensure that the monitor is at eye level. Keep the mouse near enough so as to ensure your elbow remains bent at a 90 degrees angle. Also, remember to keep things such as phones and pens within a distance of 14 to 16 inches. Your aim should be to keep your hands supported whenever you sit at your desk.

But don't stay at your desk for hours no matter how comfortable you are. Instead, you need to take frequent breaks. During the breaks, you can take brief walks to relieve muscle tension. You can also stretch your muscles gently to keep them in top form. The break will prevent you from being in the same position for long hours and give your muscles a good stretch to prevent cramping and muscle strain.

Apart from watching how you hold your body when standing and sitting, you also need to watch your posture when driving. Driving can be a stressful experience by itself. When it is combined with poor posture, it can bring you a lot of pain.

How to improve your posture when driving:

In order to maintain a good posture and avoid injuring your neck when driving, you should:

Sit properly

A good driving posture starts with the way you sit. When you sit down in your car, you should ensure that your seat is at 100 degrees. It should not be straight. It should be bent backwards just a little bit. Your hands should be at the 3 o'clock and 9 o'clock positions. As you hold the steering wheel, your hands should be relaxed and your elbows should be able to rest on the armrests comfortably.

Support your head

When it comes to the car seat, your head should be supported well. The middle part of the head should be able to rest on the headrest. This may mean making some adjustments to your car seat. If the back of your head is lower than the headrest, you will put a significant amount of strain on your neck and this will lead to neck pain. If need be, you can use a car pillow so as to be able to reach the headrest.

Make sure your back is supported

Your lower back needs to be supported when you are driving. Remember, it has a natural curve and as such, sitting on a straight seat will cause it to strain. If your vehicle has lumbar support, make sure you adjust it well so that it can fit the curve at your lower back. If your car provides no such support, you can easily rectify the situation by using a small pillow. Also, remember to adjust the car seat such that it is close to the steering well. This will prevent you from awkwardly leaning forward and staring your back and neck.

Make adjustments to your mirrors

As you drive, you'll find yourself looking into your car mirrors from time to time. If you don't place your mirrors correctly, you'll have to keep moving your head in order to see properly. This should not be the case. You need to adjust the mirror position so as to avoid moving your head when peering into the mirrors.

Avoid eyestrain

If you drive with poor vision, you won't be able to see the road ahead of you as well as you should. This will cause you to move your neck forwards in an attempt to see more clearly. If you do that, you'll place pressure on the neck muscles and this will lead to neck pain. If you strain while driving, you should go for an eye checkup to ensure you can actually see properly. Another thing you can do is keep your windshield clean. You can also make it a point to protect your eyes from harsh sunlight by using sunglasses.

Cruise

If you find yourself driving along the highway or on long stretches of a road, you can give your neck a break by employing cruise control. Cruise control does the admirable job of allowing your feet to be planted on the floor. This in turn takes some pressure off your neck and back.

Think of cruise control as you would a short break. If you're on the highway, it would be obviously difficult to get out of your vehicle and stretch your legs. But with cruise control, you let go and give your feet a break. This small break allows your muscles to relax and you'll be better for it when you take over control again.

Give yourself a break

If you are going on a long journey, you should do your research beforehand to know where you can stop for a rest. For example, if the journey is 8 hours, you can decide to stop twice within those eight hours. Once you stop, do some stretching exercises and take a short walk to loosen your muscles.

But you don't have to wait for a long journey to take a rest.

Whenever you're driving, if you feel your neck getting stiff, you can pull into the next rest stop and do some stretches to give your neck a break. Remember, neck pain can only get worse if you force yourself to remain in an uncomfortable position. If your neck is hurting, it needs a break. There is no shame in taking one.

At the end of the day, you must work on your posture if you want to improve. This starts by being conscious about the way you hold yourself. Once you are aware of what you are doing, you can make the necessary adjustments to correct your posture.

Now let's look at another thing you can do to treat neck pain.

Chapter 6: Neck Exercises

A strong neck contributes to the health of your shoulders, upper back and arms. It makes your neck more limber and loosens a tense neck. It also allows you to gain greater flexibility and get rid of pain. There are various stretching exercises you can do to loosen your neck muscles. These include:

Forward and backward tilt

In order to perform this move, you can choose to sit down or stand up. You should:

- Keep your back straight and position your head over your shoulders in a natural position. Your head should not be tilted backwards or forwards, as this is the starting point.

- Slowly move your chin towards your chest region. Once done, hold the position for 15-30 seconds and then relax and carefully move your head back up. You can gently use your index finger on your chin to push your chin towards your chest to assist you if this helps.

- Next, tilt your chin upwards towards the ceiling. The base of your skull should move towards your back. Hold the position for 10 seconds before returning to the starting point.

- Repeat the set 3-5 times and do it daily.

Side tilt

In order to do the side tilt, you should stand up straight and place your feet about hip-width apart, your arms should be by your sides. Once done, you should:

- Ensure your back is straight and that your head is over your shoulders.

- Gently move or tilt your head to the right and try to touch your right shoulders with your right ear. Once you feel the stretch, stop moving and refrain from raising your shoulders. Hold the position for 5-10 seconds before going back to the starting point.

- Gently move or tilt your head to the left side and try to touch your left shoulder with your left ear. Once you feel the stretch, hold the position for 5-10 seconds and then move back to your starting point.

- Repeat the set up to 10 times.

You don't have to complete the 10 sets. You can slowly work your way up, as you get more comfortable while doing the stretch.

Side rotation

This stretch can be done while standing or sitting. In order to do it, you should:

- Place your head over your shoulders and keep your back straight.

- Turn your head slowly towards your right shoulder. Stop when you feel a stretch in your neck and shoulder and hold the position for 15-30 seconds. You can gently use your left index finger on the left side of your jaw to assist you if this helps.

- Return your head to the starting position.

- Turn your head slowly towards your left shoulder. Stop when you feel a stretch in your neck and shoulder and proceed to hold the position for about 15 to 30 seconds. This time use your right index finger on your right jaw to gently stretch your neck rotating to the left shoulder.

- Return your head to the starting position.

- Repeat the stretch up to 10 sets.

Shoulder roll

This stretch should be done standing up. You should:

- Place your shoulders straight up and allow your hands to fall to your sides.

- Move your shoulders forward in a circle up to 6 times.

- Return to your starting point.

- Move your shoulders backwards in a circle up to 6 circles.

As you do this stretching exercise, do not move your head or neck.

Remember, the idea of doing stretching exercises is to loosen your neck and get rid of pain and tension. As you stretch, you may feel some tension. You should not move beyond the point of the stretch or try to force your neck to move more than it should. However, if you do the stretches regularly, your neck will become more flexible and in time, you'll be able to increase your range of motion without hurting yourself. Always remember to move slowly whenever you exercise your neck.

Stretching exercises should help you relieve pain but if you wish to strengthen your neck, you can go ahead and do simple exercises. Neck exercises not only improve your neck strength but they also help you to increase your range of motion. Some exercises you can do include:

Rotations

In order to do rotations, you should:

- Stand or sit in a comfortable position. Your head should be over your shoulders and your back should be straight.

- Move your head to one side as far as you can without being uncomfortable. Once done, hold the position for about 30 seconds.

- Return your head to the starting point.

- Move your head to the other side as far as you can. Hold the position for about 30 seconds.

- Repeat the exercise up to 5 times and gradually work up to 10 times.

If you are unable to hold the position for 30 seconds, don't force yourself to do it. You can gradually work up to the time as your neck gains more flexibility.

Shoulder circles

In order to do the shoulder circles, you should:

- Stand up straight and raise your shoulders straight up. Your hands should be at your sides.

- Move your shoulders in a circle one way and then return to the starting position.

- Move your shoulders in a circle in the other direction.

- Repeat the exercise up to 5 times and gradually work up to 10 times.

Resistance exercises

In order to do resistance exercises, you should:

- Stand up or sit down straight. Make sure you are comfortable before embarking on the exercise.

- Place your left hand just above your left ear on the side of your head.

- Once done, gently press your head into your left hand while keeping your head straight. The idea is to offer resistance as you stretch your neck muscles.

- Once done, return to the starting point and relax your muscles.

- Place your right hand just above your right ear on the side of your head.

- Once done, gently press your head into your right hand while keeping your hand straight. Hold the position for a few seconds.

- Repeat the exercise up to 10 times.

Head lifts

In order to do head lifts, you should:

- Lie on the floor. Your knees should be bent and your feet should be planted flat on the floor. Your hands should be by your sides on the floor.

- Once done, proceed to lift and then lower your head. You should not raise your shoulders. You are not doing sit ups. You are doing head lifts-the keyword is head. Keep your other body parts as stationary as you can.

- You can do the head lifts while lying on your stomach or on your side.

- Repeat the exercise up to 10 times. If you can't make it to 10 repetitions, start where you are comfortable and work your way towards the whole set of repetitions.

As with neck stretches, neck exercises are meant to relieve pain not add on to it. Unfortunately, when you are already in pain, it can be difficult to perform any exercises. This is why you need to exercise caution as you engage in exercise. You can talk to your physician before embarking on any exercise.

You can also make your work a bit easier by using a heating pad. Use the heating pad to warm up your joints and muscles before you embark on your stretching exercises. This will make stretching easier. Once you are done with the exercises, you can use a cold pack to reduce inflammation and allow your joints and muscles to cool down.

So far, we've seen the stretching exercises and simple exercises you can do to not only relieve but also prevent neck pain. But there is another form of exercise you can do to strengthen your neck and relieve pain. This is aerobic exercise.

Aerobic exercise

Aerobic exercise or cardio is a common workout fueled by oxygen. It keeps your heart pumping and enhances your breathing. It also increases the flow of blood to your muscles and soft tissues. This is important, as it loosens the muscles in your neck and upper back. It also works to increase your range of motion.

But there's another thing aerobic exercise does.

It releases endorphins. These act as a natural painkiller and can be quite useful in reducing neck pain. You can embark on aerobic exercises such as taking a brisk walk, exercising on the treadmill or even exercising on a stationary bike. Once you select the aerobic exercise you want, you should try to do it for at least 30 minutes to get the most out of the exercise.

Of course, if you are not used to exercising, you should pace yourself instead of overworking your muscles. It's better you exercise for 5 minutes each day instead of exercising for 1 hour and ending up in more pain because you have overextended your muscles. Also, remember to listen to your body. As we've said before, exercise is not meant to bring you pain.

When you start to exercise, your muscles may protest, especially if they have not been in regular use. You may feel your muscles stretch but this is the point where you stop doing what you're doing and hold the position. Anything beyond that can only bring you pain. Before you start to exercise, you should stretch your muscles. This will warm up your muscles and prevent you from exercising cold muscles and putting yourself at a higher risk for injury.

All in all, exercise is not only good for your general health but it is also good when it comes to relieving and preventing pain. But there are other things that can come in handy too. These are essential oils.

Chapter 7: Essential Oils To Treat Neck Pain

Essential oils have been used for centuries to provide relief from pain. They are at the forefront of aromatherapy and various types of massage therapies. It's little wonder that they can also relieve neck pain.

But that's not a fluke.

Essential oils are able to relieve pain due to their various healing properties. They have pain-relieving, analgesic and anti-inflammatory properties that are useful in getting rid of pain.

What's more, they are natural products. This means they don't have the toxins present in so many lab-made pain-relieving products. If you use them correctly, you'll benefit from their healing abilities without experiencing any side effects.

So, which essential oils can you use to treat neck pain? Well. You can use:

Basil oil

Basil oil comes in handy to soothe headaches and muscle spasms. As we've seen, one of the symptoms of neck pain is muscle spasms. These spasms can happen at night and leave you with a knotted feeling in your neck when you wake up. Basil oil is equipped with pain-relieving, anti-inflammatory, anti-viral and anti-bacterial properties that will help you find relief.

Peppermint oil

Peppermint essential is one of the most common oils used when it comes to relieving pain. Its soothing nature and mint aroma makes leaves you feeling refreshed. It can help you relieve neck pain that is brought on by things such as stress or tension. Apart from using it to massage your muscles, you can diffuse it to find relief from pain.

Frankincense oil

Frankincense essential oil is often used to treat arthritis. Arthritis in the neck is a difficult condition to live with. But frankincense oil makes it bearable as it not only reduces pain and inflammation but it also reduces stress and anxiety. What's good about frankincense is that you can apply it on your skin or inhale it directly. If you feel tension in your neck, you can easily rub some oil on the area to find relief.

Wintergreen oil

Wintergreen oil is often used in various ointments. It has that fresh mint smell that is inviting and it is often used to treat respiratory diseases. But it can also be used to treat body pain. Wintergreen oil has an aromatic property that is used to uplift the mood. If you're suffering from stress, you can use it to boost your mood and get rid of the tension in your neck muscles. But remember to dilute the oil before use, as it is quite potent.

Marjoram oil

This essential oil is full of health benefits and one of its benefits happens to be pain relief. Marjoram has antiviral, antiseptic and digestive properties that can soothe you and provide relief from pain. Its leaves are often used in the production of marjoram oil. But before using the oil, remember to test it on your skin first.

Cypress oil

When it comes to relieving pain, one essential oil you should not ignore is cypress essential oil. It has strong pain-relieving properties that can soothe tensed up muscles. Cypress oil also helps to strengthen your muscles. Thus, if you use it regularly, your muscles will be less likely to cramp. You'll be able to get rid of muscle spasms or issues associated with things like nerve pain.

Fir needle oil

Another essential oil you can use is fir needle oil. This essential oil acts as a great pain reliever. It also helps prevents infections and gets rid of cramps and aches in your muscles. Another thing it does is improve blood circulation. This enables your muscles to function properly and lessens the chances of cramping and spasms.

All these essential oils can help you relieve pain. But before they do, you need to know how to use them in order to get the best results.

How to use essential oils

There are various ways to use essential oils. You can use them in:

A relaxing bath

In order to use essential oils for a relaxing bath, you should:

- Combine an ounce of carrier oil with 12 to 15 drops of the essential oil.

- Add the mixture to the water in your tub and let it disperse evenly.

- Soak in the water to soothe away your aches and pains.

A massage

Essential oils are often used to massage various parts of the body due to their anti-inflammatory and soothing effect. Once you mix them with carrier oil, you can go ahead and massage your neck and shoulder areas.

Another thing you can do is add the essential oil to a cold or hot compress. For instance, you can add a few drops to a towel with warm water and place it on your aching muscles instead of using a plain compress to relieve pain. This way, the anti-inflammatory effects of the essential oil will combine with the soothing effects of the compress to bring you greater comfort.

A diffuser

A diffuser helps you to inhale essential oils as you go about your day. Once you select the essential oil you want to use, you can add a few drops of it to your diffuser and breathe in the scent to get the therapeutic benefits it brings. If you spend long hours at a desk, you can even purchase a USB diffuser that will dispense the essential oil as you work.

A roll-on

Another way to use essential oils is in a roll-on bottle. These bottles are convenient to use. You can easily use them several times in a day without drawing undue attention to yourself. In order to use an essential oil roll-on you should:

- Add 15 drops of your favorite essential oil to a roll-on bottle.

- Add one ounce of carrier oil to the bottle.

- Place the roller on the bottle and then proceed to seal it.

- Shake the bottle for about 30 seconds to combine the ingredients.

- Apply the essential oil to problem areas several times a day.

Yes, there are various essential oils that can help you relieve pain and you can use them in a variety of ways. But you need to be careful to only use the ones that will not irritate you. You can do a skin patch test by applying a small amount of the essential oil to your skin and waiting for 24 hours to check the results. You can also diffuse the oil in the air to see how you react to it.

Once you know which essential oils agree with you, you still have to make sure you dilute them with carrier oil before applying them topically. If you do that, you will see great results.

But apart from using essential oils, there is another thing you can do to treat neck pain. You can go on an anti-inflammatory diet. Let's see what this is about.

Chapter 8: Anti-Inflammatory Foods To Treat Neck Pain

One cause of neck pain you shouldn't dismiss is inflammation. Inflammation is supposed to be a good thing, as it is how your body guards against intruders. Unfortunately, the body can turn against itself when it is bombarded with chronic inflammation.

Think about it.

Nowadays, there are so many things that cause havoc in your body. Things like toxins, air pollutants, disease and such like things are seen as foreign invaders by your body. Your body becomes inflamed, as it fights to get rid of them. But when your body is involved in a constant battle with foreign invaders, it soon loses sight of its enemies and starts attacking everything in sight, including its own healthy cells.

When this happens, things like disease and injuries become more common. Thus, it is important to get rid of inflammation if you want to remain pain-free. You can do this by adopting an anti-inflammatory diet.

What is an anti-inflammatory diet?

Well, an anti-inflammatory diet is a diet that is high in antioxidants. One thing about inflammation is that it causes a rise in free radicals. Free radicals are highly reactive molecules that search for unpaired electrons that they can become paired with. They go as far as stealing electrons from nearby molecules and this gives birth to an imbalance known as oxidative stress. In turn, oxidative stress leads to chronic inflammation and all the health issues and pain that come with it.

Antioxidants do the important work of donating electrons that can be paired with free radicals. This neutralizes the free radicals and lessens the damage they can bring in the body. Thus, if you focus on embracing an anti-inflammatory diet, you will greatly reduce inflammation and find relief from pain and aches.

In order to start an anti-inflammatory diet, you should:

Eat more fruits and vegetables

The first thing you need to do is prioritize the consumption of fruits and vegetables. Each day, you should try to eat at least 2 servings of fruit and 3 to 5 servings of vegetables. Fruits and vegetables are great sources of antioxidants. They help fight inflammation and they also happen to be rich in nutrients.

Eat fish

Fish should be part of your diet each week. You should endeavor to eat it at least twice a week. This is because it contains omega-3 fatty acids, which happen to have great anti-inflammatory properties. A lot of people shy away from eating fish because of fear of contamination. However, if you get your fish from a reputable source, you should be okay. Go for fish such as salmon and sardines.

Use healthier fats

Trans fat or saturated fat should not be present in your diet when you are trying to fight inflammation. This is because such fats contribute to inflammation. Saturated fats found in foods such as cheese and butter are sweet and tasty but they also include more inflammatory ingredients than unsaturated fats. Unsaturated fats such as olive oil, walnuts, flaxseed and almonds are a preferable source of fat since they help fight inflammation.

Limit meats

Red meats such as beef have long been singled out as a source of inflammation. They contribute to a variety of diseases and as such, it is not advisable to consume them regularly. If you want to eat meat, you should eat lean meats such as chicken and turkey. Also, you should try as much as possible to eat organic. Factory farmed meats are usually more inflammatory than organic meats and thus, they should be limited.

If at all possible, you should create the habit of getting your protein from legumes. Instead of consuming meat each day, you can get your protein from foods such as lentils, peas, nuts or beans. These legumes are a rich source of antioxidants.

Eat whole grains

Refined grains happen to have more inflammatory properties than whole grains. As such, you should endeavor to select whole grain versions of foods such as rice, pasta, bread and oatmeal. Whole grain foods are not only less inflammatory but also more nutritious. Unfortunately, if you are used to eating refined foods, you may find the taste of whole grain foods a little 'too rich'. But don't worry. Once you continue eating such foods, you'll get used to the taste.

Avoid processed foods

Processed foods wreck havoc in your body. They are not good for you and have been linked with health issues such as obesity, heart disease and diabetes. They also happen to be highly inflammatory. This is because of the chemicals added in such foods.

In order to get the foods, look and taste a certain way, chemicals are added to them. Such foods are also often stripped down of their nutrients. Thus, they are less nutritious and more inflammatory than unprocessed foods.

In order to reduce inflammation, you should avoid prepackaged meals, processed meats such as sausage, ham and bacon, refines sugars such as candy and soda as well as baked goods. The idea is to stick to foods that are in their natural state or very near to their natural state. Foods that cause you more harm than good should not be a mainstay in your diet.

All in all, it is good to remember that there are various things you can do to find relief from pain. Don't just try out one thing. Instead, combine the various options and say goodbye to neck pain.

When Home Remedies Fail

Acupuncture

Some patient with chronic neck patient will utilize acupuncture to alleviate neck pain and stiffness. Acupuncture has been used in China for thousands of years. It involves the placement of thin needles in the skin at specific points on the body, depending on what is being treated. According to Traditional Chinese Medicine theory, acupuncture helps treat various conditions by unblocking energy (qi) so it can resume flowing naturally through its normal pathways (meridians).

Although, scientific studies have not yet confirmed the existence of qi or meridians. Some studies have found that acupuncture can stimulate biochemical changes both locally (where the needles are placed) and in the central nervous system. There are scientific theories that these biochemical changes may help pain relief for some patients.

Acupuncture treatments can vary widely based on the practitioner's training, methods and treatment strategy. Success varies from patient to patient. In most cases, the acupuncturist starts by asking about the patient's symptoms, diet, and daily routine, which may give clues about the most effective points on the body to place the needles.

Seeking Treatment with Your Doctor

Know when to seek medical treatment. There are "red flags" that should indicate you should discuss your neck pain with your doctor or train medical provider.

- Changes to your bowel or bladder

- Numbness or tingling in your arms or legs

- Recent falls

- Pain lasting longer than 6 weeks

- Fevers

- Weight loss

- Severe headaches, rashes or joint pain

- Feeling unwell, unexplained dizziness, nausea or vomiting

Neck pain may be a symptom of a more serious underlying medical condition, so it is always important to follow up with your physician or health care professional to seek guidance for your health. Don't take your health for granted.

Conclusion

We have come to the end of the book. Thank you for reading and congratulations for reading until the end.

No doubt, neck pain is not something you want to ignore. Seriously; why live in pain when you can do something to alleviate that pain? If you use the various treatments discussed in this book to get rid of neck pain and ensure that your posture is right and that you eat foods that work to prevent neck pain, you will be able to live a pain-free life and easily manage neck pain should it come up again in future.

If you found the book valuable, can you recommend it to others? One way to do that is to post a review on Amazon.

This book is for educational purposes only and is not meant to replace your doctor's advice. Always seek the advice of your physician or qualified health care provider regarding a medical condition.

Click here to leave a review for this book on Amazon!

Thank you and good luck!

www.ingramcontent.com/pod-product-compliance
Lightning Source LLC
Chambersburg PA
CBHW051235250726
48655CB00006B/2793